TRUE STRENGTH FITNESS

For Beginners

A Comprehensive Guide To Building Muscle, Burning Fat, And Achieving Peak Health With Easy-To-Follow Workouts, Nutritional Tips, And Motivational Strategies

ROBERT LUGO

CHAPTER 1 4
    Understanding True Strength 4

CHAPTER 2 11
    Foundations Of Fitness 11

CHAPTER 3 16
    Strength Training Fundamentals 16

CHAPTER 4 20
    Cardiovascular Conditioning 20

CHAPTER 5 25
    Nutrition For Strength And Health 25

CHAPTER 6 31
    Recovery And Regeneration 31

CHAPTER 7 35
    Mental Fitness And Mindfulness 35

CHAPTER 8 40
    Advanced Strength Techniques 40

CHAPTER 9 47
    Injury Prevention And Management 47

CHAPTER 10 51

Long-Term Fitness And Lifestyle 51

CHAPTER 11 55

True Strength Success Stories 55

CHAPTER 12 61

The Future Of True Strength 61

Conclusion 66

CHAPTER 1
Understanding True Strength

True strength in the context of fitness goes beyond just physical prowess. It encompasses a holistic approach that integrates physical, mental, and emotional aspects of strength. At its core, true strength is about developing not just muscles but also resilience, determination, and a positive mindset. It involves understanding the body's capabilities and limitations while striving for continuous improvement.

True strength training emphasizes functional fitness, which means training movements that mimic real-life activities. This approach helps individuals not only build muscle but also improve everyday tasks and reduce the risk of injuries. It focuses on improving overall fitness levels rather than just aesthetics, promoting longevity and quality of life.

Key principles of true strength training include progressive overload, which involves gradually increasing the intensity of workouts to stimulate muscle growth and adaptation. It also emphasizes proper form and technique to ensure safety and effectiveness. Additionally, rest and recovery are essential components to allow the body to repair and grow stronger.

Benefits of True Strength Training

The benefits of true strength training are multifaceted and extend beyond physical fitness. One of the primary advantages is increased muscle strength and endurance, which enhances performance in various physical activities and reduces the risk of injuries. It also contributes to better posture, balance, and coordination, improving overall movement efficiency.

Moreover, true strength training plays a crucial role in enhancing bone density, especially important for women and older adults to prevent osteoporosis and fractures.

It promotes a healthy body composition by reducing body fat and increasing lean muscle mass, which can positively impact metabolism and overall health.

Another significant benefit is the mental and emotional impact of true strength training. Regular exercise releases endorphins, neurotransmitters that promote feelings of happiness and well-being. It helps reduce stress, anxiety, and depression while improving cognitive function and overall mood.

Furthermore, true strength training fosters self-discipline, resilience, and confidence. Achieving fitness goals requires dedication and perseverance, which translates into other areas of life, promoting a sense of accomplishment and empowerment.

Mind-Body Connection in Fitness

The mind-body connection is a fundamental aspect of true strength training. It refers to the link between mental and emotional states and physical performance during exercise.

Cultivating a strong mind-body connection enhances overall fitness by improving focus, concentration, and awareness of movement.

Mindfulness practices such as meditation, deep breathing, and visualization are integral to developing the mind-body connection.

These techniques help individuals stay present during workouts, tune into their body's signals, and optimize performance while reducing the risk of injuries.

Additionally, the mind-body connection plays a role in regulating stress hormones like cortisol, promoting relaxation and recovery. It also enhances proprioception, the body's ability to sense its position and movements, leading to better coordination and motor control.

Incorporating mindfulness into fitness routines not only improves physical performance but also enhances mental resilience, emotional well-being, and overall quality of life. It fosters a deeper understanding of one's body, promotes self-awareness, and encourages a balanced approach to health and fitness.

Creating Reasonable Fitness Objectives

For long-term motivation and success, setting reasonable exercise objectives is crucial. True strength training emphasizes the importance of setting specific, measurable, achievable, relevant, and time-bound (SMART) goals that align with individual capabilities and aspirations.

When setting fitness goals, it's crucial to consider factors such as current fitness level, medical history, lifestyle constraints, and personal preferences. This ensures that goals are realistic and attainable, reducing the risk of burnout or injury from overtraining.

Breaking down long-term goals into smaller milestones makes progress more manageable and provides a sense of accomplishment along the way. It's essential to track progress regularly, adjust goals as needed, and celebrate achievements to stay motivated and focused.

Moreover, setting non-scale victories such as improved energy levels, better sleep, increased strength, or enhanced mood can be equally rewarding and motivating. True strength training encourages a balanced approach to goal-setting that considers both physical and mental well-being.

In conclusion, understanding true strength involves recognizing its holistic nature encompassing physical, mental, and emotional aspects. The benefits of true strength training extend beyond physical fitness to include mental resilience, emotional well-being, and overall quality of life.

The mind-body connection plays a crucial role in optimizing fitness performance while setting realistic goals is key to long-term success and motivation. Integrating these concepts into fitness routines promotes a balanced approach to health and well-being, fostering lasting changes and sustainable results.

CHAPTER 2
Foundations Of Fitness

In understanding somatic exercises for beginners, it's crucial to delve into the foundational aspects of fitness that underpin this approach.

This includes a comprehensive look at anatomy and physiology basics, the principles of exercise science, an exploration of muscle groups, and the significance of flexibility and mobility in overall fitness.

Anatomy and Physiology Basics: Anatomy refers to the study of the structure and organization of the body, while physiology focuses on how the body's systems function. For somatic exercises, a fundamental grasp of anatomy and physiology is essential. This includes understanding major body systems such as the skeletal, muscular, cardiovascular, and respiratory systems. Knowledge of skeletal structure provides insight into joint movements and limitations, which is vital for safe and effective somatic practice. Similarly, understanding muscle physiology aids in targeting specific muscle groups during exercises, promoting balanced development and injury prevention. Anatomical knowledge also extends to neurological aspects, as somatic exercises often involve mind-body connections and proprioception.

Principles of Exercise Science: Exercise science encompasses the scientific principles behind physical activity and its effects on the body. Key principles include specificity, overload, progression, adaptation, and reversibility. Specificity emphasizes that training effects are specific to the type of exercise performed, highlighting the importance of tailoring somatic exercises to individual needs and goals.

Overload involves applying sufficient stress to challenge the body and stimulate improvements, while progression entails gradually increasing intensity or complexity to promote continuous adaptation.

Understanding these principles guides the design of effective somatic exercise programs that promote gradual improvement and long-term sustainability.

Understanding Muscle Groups: Muscles play a central role in somatic exercises, as these movements often target specific muscle groups for strength, flexibility, and coordination.

Major muscle groups include the quadriceps, hamstrings, glutes, chest, back, shoulders, arms, and core muscles. Each group serves distinct functions, such as the quadriceps for knee extension, the core muscles for stability and posture, and the back muscles for spinal support.

Knowledge of muscle anatomy and function informs exercise selection and ensures comprehensive muscle engagement during somatic workouts.

This understanding also aids in preventing muscle imbalances and promoting overall muscular health.

Importance of Flexibility and Mobility: Flexibility refers to the range of motion around a joint, while mobility encompasses the ability to move freely and efficiently through various positions or movements. Both flexibility and mobility are integral components of somatic exercises, contributing to improved posture, movement quality, and injury prevention.

Flexibility allows for greater joint mobility and reduces the risk of muscle strains or joint stiffness. Incorporating stretching and mobility exercises into somatic routines enhances overall flexibility, joint health, and functional movement patterns. Understanding the role of flexibility and mobility guides the selection of exercises that promote dynamic range of motion and joint integrity, enhancing the overall effectiveness of somatic training programs.

By grounding somatic exercises in the foundational principles of fitness, including anatomy and physiology basics, exercise science principles, understanding muscle groups, and emphasizing flexibility and mobility, beginners can develop a solid framework for safe, effective, and sustainable somatic practice. This knowledge not only enhances physical performance but also promotes holistic well-being and long-term adherence to somatic training regimens.

CHAPTER 3
Strength Training Fundamentals

Strength training is a fundamental aspect of physical fitness that encompasses various exercises and techniques aimed at improving muscular strength, endurance, and overall functional capacity.

Understanding the basics of strength training is essential for beginners to establish a solid foundation and achieve long-term success in their fitness journey. This section explores key concepts such as the basics of strength training, types of resistance training, proper form and technique, and principles of progression and overload.

Strength training involves the use of resistance to induce muscular contractions, leading to increased strength, size, and endurance of muscles.

The primary goal is to challenge the muscles to adapt and grow stronger over time. Beginners often start with bodyweight exercises before progressing to using external resistance such as weights, bands, or machines. These exercises target specific muscle groups and can be performed using various techniques and equipment.

Types of resistance training include isotonic (dynamic) and isometric (static) exercises. Isotonic exercises involve movement of the muscles against resistance, such as lifting weights or performing bodyweight exercises like squats and push-ups. Isometric exercises, on the other hand, involve static muscle contractions without joint movement, such as holding a plank position or wall sit. Both types of training offer unique benefits and can be combined for a well-rounded strength training program.

Proper form and technique are crucial aspects of strength training to ensure safety, effectiveness, and optimal results. Beginners should focus on learning correct posture, alignment, and movement patterns for each exercise.

This includes maintaining a neutral spine, engaging core muscles, using a full range of motion, and avoiding jerky or excessive movements. Proper breathing techniques also play a role in enhancing performance and reducing the risk of injury during strength training.

Progression and overload principles are central to advancing in strength training and stimulating muscle growth. Progression involves gradually increasing the intensity, volume, or complexity of exercises over time to continue challenging the muscles and promoting adaptation.

This can be achieved by adding weight, increasing repetitions or sets, adjusting rest periods, or incorporating advanced variations of exercises. Overload refers to applying sufficient stress to the muscles to stimulate growth, but not to the point of causing excessive fatigue or injury. Finding the right balance of progression and overload is key to sustainable gains in strength and fitness.

Mastering the basics of strength training is essential for beginners to lay a strong foundation for their fitness journey. Understanding the types of resistance training, practicing proper form and technique, and implementing progression and overload principles are key components of a successful strength training program.

With consistent practice, guidance from qualified professionals, and a focus on gradual improvement, beginners can achieve their strength and fitness goals safely and effectively.

CHAPTER 4
Cardiovascular Conditioning

Cardiovascular conditioning is a crucial aspect of overall fitness, especially for beginners embarking on their fitness journey through somatic exercises.

Understanding the importance of cardiovascular fitness, different types of cardio workouts, heart rate training zones, and how to incorporate cardio with strength training can significantly enhance the effectiveness of a beginner's somatic exercise routine.

The efficiency with which the heart, lungs, and circulatory system function is referred to as cardiovascular fitness. work together to supply oxygen and nutrients to the muscles during physical activity. It plays a vital role in improving endurance, reducing the risk of heart disease, and enhancing overall well-being. For beginners, focusing on cardiovascular conditioning sets a solid foundation for more intense workouts and helps in achieving long-term fitness goals.

There are several types of cardio workouts suitable for beginners engaging in somatic exercises.

These include:

1. Low-Impact Cardio: Activities like walking, swimming, and cycling are gentle on the joints and ideal for beginners starting with somatic exercises. They help improve cardiovascular endurance without placing excessive stress on the body.

2. High-intensity interval training, or HIIT, alternates short bursts of high-intensity exercise with rest intervals or lower-intensity activities. It is effective in improving cardiovascular fitness, burning calories, and boosting metabolism.

3. Dance-Based Cardio: Dance workouts, such as Zumba or aerobics, combine cardio with fun and rhythm.

They are suitable for beginners looking to add variety and enjoyment to their workout routine.

4. Cardio Machines: Treadmills, elliptical trainers, and stationary bikes offer controlled environments for cardiovascular workouts. Beginners can adjust intensity levels based on their fitness level and gradually increase the challenge over time.

Understanding heart rate training zones is essential for optimizing cardio workouts. These zones are:

1. Resting Heart Rate: The heart rate when the body is at rest, typically between 60-100 beats per minute (BPM) for adults.

2. Target Heart Rate Zone: This zone represents the optimal range of heartbeats per minute during

exercise to achieve cardiovascular benefits. It is usually calculated based on age, resting heart rate, and fitness goals.

3. Maximum Heart Rate: The highest heart rate an individual can achieve during intense exercise.

It is often estimated using formulas like 220 minus age.

Incorporating cardio with strength training is a strategic approach to comprehensive fitness. Combining these two forms of exercise offers a balanced workout routine that enhances cardiovascular health, builds strength, and improves overall body composition. Beginners can integrate cardio into their somatic exercise regimen by:

1. Warm-up and Cool-down: Start and end each workout session with a brief cardio activity, such as brisk walking or cycling, to prepare the body for exercise and aid in recovery.

2. Circuit Training: Create circuits that include both strength exercises and cardio intervals. For example, perform a set of bodyweight squats followed by a minute of jumping jacks or mountain climbers.

3. Interval Training: Alternate between strength exercises and cardio bursts within the same workout. This approach keeps the heart rate elevated while engaging different muscle groups.

4. Cross-Training: Incorporate a variety of cardio activities throughout the week to prevent boredom, challenge different muscle groups, and improve overall fitness levels.

By understanding the importance of cardiovascular fitness, exploring various types of cardio workouts, mastering heart rate training zones, and seamlessly integrating cardio with strength training, beginners can enhance their somatic exercise experience and achieve holistic fitness benefits.

CHAPTER 5
Nutrition For Strength And Health

Nutrition plays a pivotal role in achieving optimal health and fitness, especially when combined with somatic exercises designed for beginners. Understanding the fundamentals of nutrition is crucial for enhancing strength, promoting recovery, and sustaining overall well-being.

This section delves into the intricate interplay between nutrition and somatic exercise for beginners, covering essential concepts such as the role of nutrition in fitness, macronutrients and micronutrients, meal planning for fitness goals, and the significance of hydration and recovery nutrition.

The role of nutrition in fitness is multifaceted and goes beyond mere calorie counting.

It encompasses providing the body with essential nutrients to support muscle growth, repair tissues, maintain energy levels, and regulate various bodily functions.

For beginners embarking on somatic exercises, a balanced diet rich in macronutrients (carbohydrates, proteins, and fats) and micronutrients (vitamins and minerals) is imperative. Macronutrients serve as the building blocks for muscle tissue, fueling workouts and aiding in post-exercise recovery. Proteins, in particular, play a crucial role in muscle repair and synthesis, making them essential for individuals engaging in strength-focused somatic exercises.

Understanding macronutrients and their impact on fitness is key to optimizing performance and achieving desired outcomes. Carbohydrates serve as the primary energy source during workouts, replenishing glycogen stores and sustaining endurance. For beginners, incorporating complex carbohydrates such as whole grains, fruits, and vegetables ensures sustained energy levels throughout somatic exercise sessions.

Proteins, on the other hand, are essential for muscle repair and growth, making them indispensable for individuals focusing on strength and muscle development through somatic exercises.

Lean sources of protein such as poultry, fish, legumes, and dairy products should be included in the diet to support muscle recovery and adaptation.

Micronutrients, although required in smaller quantities, play a crucial role in supporting overall health and fitness. Vitamins and minerals act as co-factors in numerous metabolic processes, aiding in energy production, immune function, and recovery. Incorporating a variety of colorful fruits and vegetables ensures adequate intake of micronutrients, promoting overall well-being and enhancing the body's resilience during somatic exercise training.

Meal planning tailored to fitness goals is a strategic approach to optimize nutrition for strength and health.

For beginners engaging in somatic exercises, meal timing, and composition can significantly impact performance and recovery. Pre-workout meals should focus on providing easily digestible carbohydrates for immediate energy, while post-workout meals should prioritize protein intake to facilitate muscle repair and recovery.

Planning meals that strike a balance between macronutrients ensures sustained energy levels, promotes muscle growth, and supports overall fitness progression.

Hydration is another critical aspect of nutrition for strength and health, especially in the context of somatic exercises. Proper hydration is essential for maintaining electrolyte balance, regulating body temperature, and supporting optimal muscle function. Beginners should aim to stay adequately hydrated throughout the day, particularly before, during, and after somatic exercise sessions. Consuming water-rich foods such as fruits and vegetables, along with regular water intake, promotes hydration and aids in recovery post-exercise.

Recovery nutrition plays a pivotal role in the effectiveness of somatic exercise programs for beginners. Post-exercise nutrition should focus on replenishing glycogen stores, supporting muscle repair, and minimizing fatigue.

Including a combination of carbohydrates and proteins in post-exercise meals or snacks accelerates recovery, reduces muscle soreness, and prepares the body for subsequent workouts. Nutrient-dense foods such as lean proteins, whole grains, fruits, and vegetables are ideal choices for promoting recovery and overall health in individuals engaging in somatic exercises.

nutrition is a cornerstone of strength and health, particularly for beginners exploring somatic exercises.

By understanding the role of nutrition in fitness, optimizing macronutrient and micronutrient intake, planning meals tailored to fitness goals, prioritizing hydration, and emphasizing recovery nutrition, beginners can enhance their performance, support muscle growth, and sustain overall well-being throughout their somatic exercise journey.

CHAPTER 6
Recovery And Regeneration

Recovery and regeneration are fundamental aspects of any fitness program, especially when it comes to somatic exercises for beginners. Understanding the importance of rest and recovery, optimizing sleep quality, employing active recovery techniques, and managing stress are key components of achieving optimal performance and long-term success in fitness endeavors.

Rest and recovery play a crucial role in the body's adaptation to exercise. When engaging in somatic exercises, beginners often focus on the intensity and frequency of workouts but may overlook the necessity of adequate rest. Rest allows the body to repair and rebuild muscle tissues that undergo stress during exercise. It also replenishes energy stores and allows for the removal of metabolic waste products, contributing to overall recovery and performance enhancement.

Sleep quality significantly impacts fitness outcomes and overall well-being. During sleep, the body undergoes essential processes such as tissue repair, hormone regulation, and memory consolidation. For beginners in somatic exercises, prioritizing sufficient and quality sleep is paramount. Research suggests that inadequate sleep can lead to impaired cognitive function, increased stress levels, and reduced exercise performance. Therefore, establishing good sleep hygiene practices, such as maintaining a consistent sleep schedule, creating a conducive sleep environment, and practicing relaxation techniques before bedtime, can positively impact fitness progress.

Active recovery techniques complement rest and sleep in promoting optimal recovery. Unlike passive rest, active recovery involves engaging in low-intensity activities that facilitate blood flow, muscle relaxation, and joint mobility. Examples of active recovery for somatic exercise beginners may include gentle stretching, walking, yoga, or swimming.

These activities promote circulation, enhance flexibility, and alleviate muscle soreness, aiding in faster recovery between workouts. Incorporating active recovery sessions into a weekly exercise routine can improve overall recovery efficiency and reduce the risk of overtraining.

Stress management is integral to optimizing performance and promoting recovery in somatic exercise beginners. Chronic stress can negatively impact physical and mental well-being, leading to increased muscle tension, fatigue, and compromised immune function.

Effective stress management techniques, such as mindfulness meditation, deep breathing exercises, progressive muscle relaxation, and engaging in hobbies or social activities, can help mitigate the negative effects of stress on the body.

By reducing stress levels, individuals can enhance their ability to recover from workouts, maintain motivation, and sustain long-term adherence to their fitness goals.

Recovery and regeneration are essential pillars of success in somatic exercises for beginners. Prioritizing rest and recovery, optimizing sleep quality, incorporating active recovery techniques, and managing stress effectively contribute to overall performance enhancement, injury prevention, and long-term fitness success.

By understanding and implementing these concepts, beginners can establish a solid foundation for their fitness journey and achieve sustainable progress in their somatic exercise practices.

CHAPTER 7
Mental Fitness And Mindfulness

Mental fitness and mindfulness play crucial roles in the journey of somatic exercises for beginners. Understanding the psychology of fitness motivation, mastering goal setting and visualization techniques, incorporating mindfulness practices into workouts, and overcoming mental barriers are all essential aspects that contribute to a successful and sustainable somatic exercise routine.

Psychology of Fitness Motivation

Motivation is a complex psychological phenomenon that drives behavior. In the context of fitness, understanding what motivates individuals to engage in somatic exercises is fundamental. Motivation can stem from various sources, such as intrinsic factors like personal goals, values, and enjoyment of the activity, or extrinsic factors like external rewards or social approval.

One psychological theory often applied to fitness motivation is Self-Determination Theory (SDT). SDT posits that motivation can be intrinsic (arising from internal desires and values) or extrinsic (driven by external rewards or pressures). For somatic exercises, fostering intrinsic motivation is key to long-term adherence.

This can be achieved by helping individuals connect their fitness goals to their core values, providing autonomy in exercise choices, and creating a supportive environment that nurtures a sense of competence and relatedness.

Goal Setting and Visualization

Setting clear and realistic goals is a cornerstone of effective fitness programming. In the context of somatic exercises, goals can range from improving flexibility and mobility to reducing stress and enhancing overall well-being.

Goal setting should follow the SMART criteria: specific, measurable, achievable, relevant, and time-bound.

Visualization is a powerful mental technique that can enhance motivation and performance.

By mentally rehearsing the successful completion of exercises, individuals can strengthen neural pathways associated with movement patterns, boost confidence, and reduce anxiety. Incorporating visualization exercises into somatic workouts can help beginners build a positive mindset and stay focused on their goals.

Mindfulness Practices for Fitness

Mindfulness involves paying attention to the present moment with a non-judgmental awareness. In the context of fitness, mindfulness practices can enhance the mind-body connection, improve exercise technique, and increase overall enjoyment. Beginners can benefit from mindfulness techniques such as mindful breathing, body scans, and mindful movement during somatic exercises.

Mindfulness also plays a role in stress reduction and emotional regulation, which are crucial for maintaining consistency in exercise routines.

By cultivating mindfulness skills, individuals can better manage stressors that may interfere with their fitness journey and develop resilience in the face of challenges.

Overcoming Mental Barriers

Everyone encounters mental barriers on their fitness journey. These barriers can manifest as self-doubt, fear of failure, lack of confidence, or resistance to change. Overcoming these barriers requires a combination of self-awareness, self-compassion, and strategic coping strategies.

Cognitive-behavioral techniques, such as cognitive restructuring and reframing negative thoughts, can help individuals challenge limiting beliefs and adopt a more positive mindset.

Building self-efficacy through progressive goal achievement and celebrating small victories can boost confidence and motivation.

Creating a supportive community and seeking guidance from experienced practitioners or mental health professionals can also provide valuable resources for overcoming mental barriers and staying committed to somatic exercises.

Mental fitness and mindfulness are integral components of a holistic approach to somatic exercises for beginners.

By understanding the psychology of fitness motivation, mastering goal-setting and visualization techniques, incorporating mindfulness practices, and overcoming mental barriers, individuals can cultivate a positive mindset and sustainably integrate somatic exercises into their lives.

CHAPTER 8
Advanced Strength Techniques

Advanced strength techniques refer to strategies used to enhance muscle strength, endurance, and overall physical performance beyond basic exercises. These techniques often involve manipulating variables such as intensity, volume, frequency, and rest periods to stimulate greater adaptations in the body.

One of the key principles in advanced strength training is progressive overload, which involves gradually increasing the demands placed on the muscles over time to promote continuous improvement.

One advanced strength technique commonly used is supersets, where two exercises targeting different muscle groups are performed back-to-back with minimal rest in between. This technique helps to maximize workout efficiency and intensity, leading to greater muscle fatigue and growth.

Another technique is drop sets, where the weight is reduced after reaching muscle failure to extend the set and induce further muscle stimulation.

Cluster sets are another advanced technique involving short rest intervals within a set, allowing for higher intensity and greater overall workload. This method is particularly effective for improving muscular endurance and metabolic conditioning. Additionally, techniques like eccentric training, where the emphasis is placed on the lowering phase of an exercise, can be used to enhance muscle strength and control.

Periodization and Training Cycles

Periodization is a systematic approach to organizing training into distinct phases or cycles to optimize performance and prevent overtraining.

It involves manipulating variables such as intensity, volume, and rest to ensure progressive improvements while minimizing the risk of injury and burnout. A typical periodization model includes phases such as the preparatory phase, strength phase, power phase, and maintenance phase.

The preparatory phase focuses on building a foundation of general fitness and addressing any weaknesses or imbalances. This phase often includes lower-intensity workouts with higher repetitions and lighter weights to improve endurance and technique. The strength phase follows, where the emphasis shifts to heavier weights and lower repetitions to increase muscle strength and size.

The power phase incorporates explosive movements and plyometric exercises to develop speed, agility, and power. This phase is crucial for athletes and individuals seeking to improve athletic performance.

Finally, the maintenance phase aims to sustain gains made during previous phases while allowing for recovery and preventing overtraining.

Training cycles within periodization can vary in duration, with shorter cycles (microcycles) focusing on weekly or bi-weekly variations in intensity and volume, and longer cycles (mesocycles) spanning several weeks or months to address specific training goals.

Advanced Strength Training Methods

In addition to traditional strength training exercises such as squats, deadlifts, and bench presses, advanced strength training methods involve specialized techniques and equipment to challenge the body in new ways. One method is the use of resistance bands or chains to add variable resistance throughout an exercise, increasing the difficulty during the concentric phase.

Another advanced method is isometric training, where muscles are contracted without joint movement, leading to improvements in static strength and stability. Isometric exercises can be incorporated into a routine to target specific muscle groups and improve overall body control. Additionally, advanced machines and equipment like the Smith machine, cable machines, and kettlebells offer unique training opportunities for advanced strength development.

Power and Plyometric Training

Power training focuses on developing explosive strength and speed through dynamic movements and high-intensity exercises. Plyometric training, a subset of power training, involves rapid stretching and contracting of muscles to improve muscular power and reactive strength.

Examples of plyometric exercises include box jumps, medicine ball throws, and depth jumps.

These exercises enhance neuromuscular coordination and fast-twitch muscle fiber recruitment, leading to improvements in athletic performance and agility. Incorporating power and plyometric training into a somatic exercise program can benefit individuals looking to improve their speed, explosiveness, and overall athletic ability.

Functional Fitness and Real-World Applications

Functional fitness emphasizes exercises and movements that mimic real-life activities and improve overall functional capacity. This approach focuses on enhancing mobility, flexibility, stability, and strength in a way that translates to everyday tasks and activities. Functional exercises often involve multi-joint movements and engage multiple muscle groups simultaneously.

Examples of functional exercises include squats, lunges, kettlebell swings, and farmer's carries. These exercises not only improve physical strength but also promote better posture, balance, and coordination. Integrating functional fitness into a somatic exercise program can help individuals develop a strong foundation of movement patterns that apply to daily life, sports, and recreational activities.

Overall, incorporating advanced strength techniques, periodization, power training, and functional fitness principles into a somatic exercise program can provide beginners with a well-rounded and effective approach to improving their overall physical fitness, performance, and functional capacity. These strategies can be tailored to individual needs and goals, making them valuable tools for long-term success in fitness and wellness.

CHAPTER 9
Injury Prevention And Management

Injury prevention and management are critical aspects of any fitness program, including somatic exercises for beginners. Understanding common fitness injuries, implementing prehabilitation exercises, managing post-injury rehabilitation, and prioritizing safety and risk management in training are fundamental pillars for ensuring a safe and effective somatic exercise regimen.

Common fitness injuries encompass a range of conditions that can occur during physical activity. These may include strains, sprains, tendonitis, stress fractures, and overuse injuries. Beginners are particularly susceptible to these injuries due to factors such as inadequate warm-up, poor technique, overexertion, or lack of proper conditioning. Educating beginners about these potential injuries and how to prevent them is crucial for their long-term well-being.

Prehabilitation exercises, often referred to as prehab, are proactive measures aimed at reducing the risk of injury. These exercises focus on strengthening muscles, improving flexibility, enhancing joint stability, and correcting movement patterns.

For somatic exercises, prehab exercises may involve movements that increase body awareness, improve posture, and enhance overall mobility. By incorporating prehabilitation into a beginner's routine, they can better prepare their bodies for the demands of somatic exercises and reduce the likelihood of injuries.

In the event of an injury, effective post-injury rehabilitation is essential for recovery and returning to regular activity safely. Rehabilitation protocols for somatic exercise injuries may involve a combination of rest, targeted exercises to promote healing and restore function, manual therapy techniques, and gradual reintroduction to physical activity.

Beginners must seek professional guidance from healthcare providers or qualified fitness professionals to ensure proper rehabilitation and prevent exacerbation of injuries.

Safety and risk management in training are foundational principles that underpin the entire somatic exercise program. This includes creating a safe exercise environment, providing clear instructions and demonstrations, emphasizing proper form and technique, monitoring intensity levels, and encouraging rest and recovery.

Beginners should be educated on safety protocols, such as using appropriate equipment, listening to their bodies, avoiding pushing through pain, and seeking guidance when unsure. By prioritizing safety in training, beginners can engage in somatic exercises with confidence and minimize the risk of injuries.

Overall, injury prevention and management are integral components of a successful somatic exercise program for beginners.

By addressing common fitness injuries, implementing prehabilitation exercises, managing post-injury rehabilitation effectively, and prioritizing safety and risk management in training, beginners can enjoy the benefits of somatic exercises while minimizing the potential risks associated with physical activity.

CHAPTER 10
Long-Term Fitness And Lifestyle

Long-term fitness is a journey that extends beyond short-lived goals or fleeting motivations.

It encompasses a holistic approach to health and well-being, integrating physical, mental, and emotional aspects of wellness. For beginners embarking on a somatic exercise journey, understanding the principles of long-term fitness is crucial for sustained progress and overall lifestyle enhancement.

Sustainable Fitness Habits

Sustainability in fitness revolves around adopting practices that are not only effective in the short term but also maintainable over extended periods. Somatic exercises for beginners offer a unique avenue to cultivate sustainable fitness habits. Unlike quick-fix solutions or intense workout regimes that can lead to burnout, somatic exercises emphasize mindful movement, body awareness, and gradual progression.

This approach encourages individuals to listen to their bodies, respect their limits, and adjust their routines accordingly, fostering a sustainable fitness mindset.

Lifestyle Changes for Health

Incorporating somatic exercises into one's lifestyle often prompts broader health-related changes. This may include adjustments in daily activities, posture awareness, ergonomic considerations in workspaces, and mindful movement practices in everyday tasks.

By integrating somatic principles into lifestyle habits, individuals can experience enhanced mobility, reduced stress, improved posture, and a heightened sense of overall well-being.

These lifestyle changes go beyond mere exercise routines, creating a holistic foundation for long-term health benefits.

Fitness for Different Life Stages

Fitness needs evolve throughout life stages, from youth to older adulthood. Somatic exercises cater to this diversity by offering adaptable routines that suit varying physical abilities and goals.

For beginners, somatic practices provide a gentle introduction to movement that can be tailored to accommodate age-related considerations, such as joint health, flexibility, and balance. As individuals progress through different life stages, somatic exercises can be modified to address changing needs, ensuring continuous improvement and vitality.

Building a Supportive Fitness Community

A supportive fitness community plays a pivotal role in sustaining long-term fitness endeavors. Engaging with like-minded individuals who share an interest in somatic exercises fosters motivation, accountability, and camaraderie. Online forums, social media groups, local classes, and workshops provide avenues for beginners to connect with peers, share experiences, seek guidance, and celebrate achievements. This sense of community not only enhances the enjoyment of somatic practices but also reinforces commitment to long-term fitness goals.

Long-term fitness and lifestyle encompass sustainable habits, lifestyle changes for health, fitness across different life stages, and the importance of building a supportive fitness community. Incorporating somatic exercises into daily life fosters a holistic approach to wellness, promoting physical, mental, and emotional well-being throughout one's fitness journey.

CHAPTER 11
True Strength Success Stories

True Strength Success Stories are not just tales of physical transformation but narratives that delve into the depth of human resilience, determination, and the power of overcoming challenges.

These stories are not just about achieving fitness goals; they are about embracing a journey of self-discovery, mental fortitude, and the unwavering spirit to succeed. Let's explore the essence of True Strength Success Stories through inspirational tales, heartfelt testimonials, insightful case studies, lessons learned, and the joy of celebrating milestones and achievements.

Inspirational Stories of Transformation

True Strength Success Stories often begin with a spark of inspiration, a moment of realization that propels individuals towards a path of change. These stories showcase the remarkable transformation journeys of people from all walks of life. From overcoming chronic pain to reclaiming lost mobility, each story reflects the indomitable human spirit. These narratives inspire others to believe in their potential, showing that with dedication and perseverance, incredible transformations are possible.

Consider the story of Sarah, a busy professional juggling work and family responsibilities. Struggling with weight gain and low energy, she felt trapped in a cycle of stress and unhealthy habits.

However, Sarah's determination to prioritize her well-being sparked a transformational journey. Through consistent exercise, mindful eating, and a supportive community, Sarah not only shed excess weight but also regained her confidence and zest for life.

Her story serves as a beacon of hope for those facing similar challenges, showing that it's never too late to embark on a journey toward better health and happiness.

Testimonials and Case Studies

Testimonials play a pivotal role in True Strength Success Stories, offering firsthand accounts of the impact of fitness and wellness journeys.

These testimonials go beyond mere words; they embody real experiences, struggles, triumphs, and transformations. Hearing from individuals who have walked the path of fitness and witnessed tangible changes in their lives adds credibility and relatability to the narrative.

Take John's testimonial, for instance. A former athlete who struggled with post-retirement weight gain and loss of motivation, John found solace and renewed purpose in a structured fitness program. Through consistent training, nutritional guidance, and mentorship, John not only regained his physical strength but also rediscovered his passion for an active lifestyle. His testimonial resonates with others facing similar transitions, offering insights into the transformative power of disciplined training and mindset shifts.

Lessons Learned from Successful Journeys

Behind every True Strength Success Story lies a tapestry of lessons learned. These lessons encapsulate the wisdom gained from challenges, setbacks, and moments of triumph. They serve as guiding principles for others embarking on their fitness and wellness journeys, offering valuable insights and strategies for sustainable success.

One of the key lessons learned is the importance of consistency and perseverance. True transformations don't happen overnight; they require dedication, patience, and a long-term commitment to healthy habits. Additionally, the value of community and support cannot be overstated.

Surrounding oneself with like-minded individuals, whether in a gym setting or virtual community, fosters accountability, motivation, and shared growth.

Celebrating Milestones and Achievements

True Strength Success Stories are incomplete without moments of celebration and acknowledgment. These milestones, whether big or small, represent significant achievements along the journey. Celebrations serve as reminders of progress made, obstacles overcome, and goals achieved, fueling motivation and resilience for the road ahead.

Imagine a community fitness event where participants showcase their progress, share success stories, and celebrate achievements together. From completing a first 5K run to mastering advanced yoga poses, each milestone is met with applause, encouragement, and a sense of collective pride. These celebrations not only honor individual accomplishments but also inspire others to set and pursue their own fitness goals with passion and determination.

True Strength Success Stories embody the transformative power of resilience, determination, and the human spirit.

Through inspirational tales of transformation, heartfelt testimonials, lessons learned, and celebrations of milestones, these stories inspire and empower individuals to embark on their journeys of health, wellness, and personal growth.

CHAPTER 12
The Future Of True Strength

The future of true strength encompasses a broad spectrum of evolving concepts and practices that are reshaping the landscape of fitness and wellness. As our understanding of human physiology deepens and technology advances, the possibilities for achieving optimal physical and mental health continue to expand.

 In this discussion, we'll explore key trends and innovations in fitness, the integration of technology with fitness, the environmental and social impact of fitness, and the importance of advocacy for health and wellness.

Trends and Innovations in Fitness The fitness industry is constantly evolving, driven by trends that reflect changing consumer preferences and scientific advancements. One prominent trend is the shift towards holistic approaches to fitness, where emphasis is placed not only on physical strength but also on mental well-being, emotional balance, and overall quality of life. This holistic view has led to the rise of practices like somatic exercises, which focus on enhancing body awareness, improving movement patterns, and reducing stress through mindful movement.

Another significant trend is the increasing popularity of functional fitness, which emphasizes movements and exercises that mimic real-life activities and improve everyday functionality.

This trend aligns well with somatic exercises, as both emphasize the importance of movement quality, mobility, and joint stability in addition to traditional strength training.

Innovations in fitness technology have also made a significant impact, with the development of wearable devices, fitness apps, and virtual training platforms. These technologies not only track and monitor fitness progress but also provide personalized workout plans, real-time feedback, and virtual coaching, making fitness more accessible and engaging for beginners.

Integrating Technology with Fitness The integration of technology with fitness has revolutionized how beginners approach their fitness journeys. Wearable devices such as fitness trackers and smartwatches provide valuable data on metrics like heart rate, calories burned, and sleep quality, empowering beginners to make informed decisions about their health and fitness routines. Fitness apps offer a wide range of workout programs, from beginner-friendly routines to advanced training plans, catering to diverse fitness goals and preferences.

Virtual reality (VR) and augmented reality (AR) technologies are also being integrated into fitness experiences, allowing beginners to engage in immersive workout sessions from the comfort of their homes. Virtual fitness classes, interactive training simulations, and gamified workout challenges provide a dynamic and interactive approach to fitness that motivates beginners to stay consistent and enjoy their workouts.

Environmental and Social Impact of Fitness The impact of fitness extends beyond individual health benefits to encompass environmental and social considerations. As awareness of environmental sustainability grows, there is a growing emphasis on eco-friendly fitness practices, such as outdoor workouts, sustainable gym equipment, and eco-conscious fitness apparel.

Beginners are encouraged to explore outdoor activities like hiking, cycling, and group fitness classes in natural settings, promoting a deeper connection with nature and a more sustainable approach to fitness.

Social impact is also a crucial aspect of fitness, as it fosters community engagement, support, and inclusivity. Fitness initiatives that promote diversity, equity, and accessibility ensure that everyone, regardless of background or ability, has the opportunity to participate and thrive in fitness activities.

Community-based fitness programs, charity runs, and fitness events that support social causes contribute to a sense of belonging and collective well-being among beginners and fitness enthusiasts alike.

Advocacy for Health and Wellness Advocacy plays a vital role in promoting health and wellness initiatives, and raising awareness about the benefits of regular exercise, balanced nutrition, and mental well-being. Health advocacy organizations, fitness professionals, and community leaders collaborate to educate beginners about the importance of prioritizing their health, seeking professional guidance, and adopting sustainable lifestyle habits.

Empowering beginners with knowledge, resources, and support networks empowers them to take ownership of their health and make positive choices that contribute to long-term well-being. Advocacy efforts also focus on breaking down barriers to fitness, such as affordability, accessibility, and cultural stigmas, to ensure that everyone has equal opportunities to lead healthy and fulfilling lives.

In conclusion, the future of true strength in fitness encompasses a holistic approach that integrates trends and innovations, leverages technology for accessibility and engagement, considers environmental and social impact, and advocates for health and wellness on individual and community levels. By embracing these concepts, beginners can embark on transformative fitness journeys that not only build physical strength but also enhance overall well-being and quality of life.

Conclusion

Congratulations on completing your journey through True Strength Fitness! You've delved into the core principles of fitness, unlocking the secrets to a healthier, stronger you. As you reflect on the chapters you've explored, remember that true strength isn't just about physical prowess—it's about a holistic approach to wellness that encompasses mind, body, and spirit.

In your quest for understanding True Strength, you've uncovered the profound benefits that come with it. From the mind-body connection that fuels your workouts to the realistic goals you've set for yourself, every step has been a building block towards a more resilient and empowered version of yourself.

Foundations of Fitness have been laid, with a deep dive into anatomy, exercise science, and the crucial role of flexibility and mobility. You've honed your Strength Training Fundamentals, mastering proper form and progression techniques that ensure safe and effective workouts.

Cardiovascular Conditioning has become second nature, blending seamlessly with your strength training to enhance overall fitness. And let's not forget the vital role of Nutrition, where you've learned to fuel your body for optimal performance and recovery.

Recovery and Regeneration have become your allies, understanding the importance of rest, sleep, and stress management in your fitness journey. Mental Fitness and Mindfulness techniques have empowered you to overcome obstacles and stay motivated, while Advanced Strength Techniques have taken your workouts to new heights.

Injury Prevention and Management are now second nature, as you've armed yourself with knowledge and prehabilitation strategies to stay safe. Looking towards Long-Term Fitness and Lifestyle, you've embraced sustainable habits and built a supportive community that fuels your progress.

Through True Strength Success Stories, you've drawn inspiration from others' journeys, celebrating milestones and achievements along the way. And as you look to the future of True Strength, you stand at the forefront of fitness innovation, integrating technology and advocating for health and wellness.

Your True Strength journey doesn't end here—it's a lifelong commitment to your well-being and vitality. So keep pushing boundaries, embracing challenges, and living your best life. Your True Strength is not just a destination; it's a way of life.

www.ingramcontent.com/pod-product-compliance
Lightning Source LLC
Chambersburg PA
CBHW050239230526
45470CB00005B/2028